I0767907

By

Kelly Schweiger

This is a work of creative nonfiction. Some parts have been fictionalized in varying degrees for various purposes.

Copyright © **Kelly Schweiger**, 2024

Kelly Schweiger

Our Journey Together:

Nurturing Understanding in Children

When a Loved One Faces Chronic Illness

Table of Contents

Disclaimer

Our Journey Together: Nurturing Understanding in Children When a Loved One Faces Chronic Illness Start a moving journey of love, strength, and kindness in "Our Journey Together." This book was written to help families trying to talk to their kids about a loved one's long-term sickness. While I am not a doctor or medical professional, I do have several incurable and chronic conditions. As the pages turn, I hope you will find a wealth of understanding insights, age-appropriate techniques, and powerful stories to unite people and help them understand each other. I hope to help address kids' fears, misunderstandings, and worries by using customized methods that work for various age groups. Having open conversations with your family is a vital part of this process. I wrote this hoping to look at ways to create a feeling of safety, use language that is appropriate for the person's age, and deal with the mental and emotional effects of having a chronic illness. Families are shown how to include children in conversations about illnesses and given practical tools and ways to work together. The guide also talks about staying stable and gives helpful advice on keeping things as normal as possible while meeting medical needs. Engaging drills and activities are added to help create a supportive family setting that builds stronger bonds and endurance.

In "Our Journey Together," the power of understanding and kindness to change things is central. Families find a wide range of activities meant to bring them closer together by building a web of shared experiences and understanding. As the trip goes on, the guide answers the kids' questions and explains why it's essential for the whole family to be strong. The most important lessons are summed up, and families are given ongoing support and tools to help them on their unique journey. People dealing with a loved one's chronic sickness can turn to "Our Journey Together" as a reliable friend, a source of inspiration, and a road plan. This book shows how strong family bonds can be. I hope it gives comfort, advice, and hope to families who are starting the long road of knowing each other while dealing with a chronic illness.

Chapter 1: Introduction

Explaining a loved one's chronic illness to children.

When trying to understand and deal with a loved one's long-term illness, one of the most challenging but most important things is describing the situation to children. Children are naturally sensitive and interested, so it's essential to approach the subject with care, understanding, and language that is right for their age. This chapter talks about how to introduce the idea of figuring out a loved one's long-term illness to children in a meaningful and helpful way. It also advises on how to communicate effectively.

Families that have someone with a chronic illness often have to deal with a lot of problems. Parents and other carers often don't know how to explain these diseases to their children. In the first part of this chapter, we'll talk about how to recognize the emotional and mental effects of chronic illnesses on the person who has them and their family. It will stress how important it is to create a safe and open space for talking about these things with kids since these talks are crucial for developing their knowledge and mental health. When discussing a chronic illness with your family, it's imperative to understand how they usually talk to each other. All families are unique, and so is the way they communicate with one another. This part will talk about the different roles that family members play in this challenging process, focusing on how important it is to present a united front and send clear messages. It will also talk about the problems that might come up, like how kids might behave based on their age, what they might think, or their fears.

To successfully explain a loved one's chronic sickness, it is crucial to take the mystery out of the idea itself. This part will discuss how to define and speak about chronic illnesses with kids in a way that is right for their age, using simple words and metaphors they can understand. It will also talk about how important it is to create an environment where questions are accepted, and curiosity is embraced so kids can understand the illness without being too overwhelmed. There are different ways that kids can react emotionally when they learn that a loved one has a long-term sickness. This part of the chapter will talk about common emotional responses, like confusion, sadness, or worry, and give parents and other carers tips on how to deal with these feelings healthily. It will show how important it is to validate kids' feelings while reassuring and helping them.

As we come to the end of this part, we want to stress that the first talk about a loved one's long-term illness is only the start. It is the start of conversations that will continue as the kids get older. We'll discuss ways to keep the lines of communication open and change how you explain things based on the child's growth stage. This will set the stage for the parts about age-specific issues.

Emotional challenges families may encounter

Family members of someone with a chronic sickness have to deal with a lot of emotional issues and problems that go beyond the physical symptoms of the disease. This chapter goes into detail about the many mental problems that families may face when dealing with a loved one's long-term sickness. Feelings significantly impact how families work and people's health, from the original shock to the long-term effects. He First Shock and Denying Sometimes, when a family member is diagnosed with a long-term illness, they are shocked and upset. The first reveal can be too much to handle, making people feel many things, including shock, fear, and doubt. Family members may be having a hard time with how their lives were suddenly turned upside down, wondering if things are fair, and trying to figure out what the illness means. During the early stages of a chronic sickness, people often feel many different emotions. This part discusses how people deal with and get through these feelings.

Grief and Loss: Getting Rid of the Emotional Stuff Chronic sickness brings about sadness and loss for the person who has it and their family. This part of the chapter talks about the complicated feelings that come with losing health, routine, and the future you had planned. Families can go through different stages of grief, such as denial, anger, bargaining, sadness, and acceptance. Understanding and accepting these feelings is essential so everyone in the family can talk about their thoughts without fear of being judged, which affects how families work. A person with a chronic illness can change the way their family works in significant ways. Things like roles and tasks can change, and the balance of power can be upset. This part talks about how these changes can cause mental stress that can lead to arguments or feelings of being alone. By looking at how family connections work together, we hope to learn how to make people more resilient and able to adapt so that families can deal with these changes with understanding and care. Living with fear and anxiety: not knowing what will happen People who have a chronic illness often feel like they don't know what the future holds. Families may be worried about how the illness will get worse, how it will affect their finances, and how it will affect their daily lives. This part of the chapter discusses the mental effects of constant uncertainty and gives ways to deal with stress and build strength. It also talks about how important it is for family members to talk to each other openly to ease worries and create a support system.

1: Burnout and compassion fatigue in carers

The mental issues can be especially hard for family members who are taking care of others. Caring for someone else while also taking care of your mental health is a tricky thing to do. This part discusses carer burnout and compassion fatigue to help you understand how emotionally worn-out carers may feel. To keep carers from getting burned out and improve their general health, strategies for self-care and the value of getting help from others are discussed—stigma and Being Left Out of Society. People who have a chronic illness may also have to deal with social stigmas and false beliefs. Some families may feel alone as they try to navigate a world that doesn't fully understand or care about their situation. This part talks about the mental problems that come up because of how other people see you and gives you tips on how to make friends, teach others, and feel like you fit.

Building up emotional strength

As we wrap up this part, we want to stress how important it is for families to build mental strength. Families can develop ways to deal with mental problems, improve communication, and build support by recognizing and talking about them head-on. This strength helps people deal with the ongoing mental challenges of chronic sickness, creating an atmosphere of understanding, empathy, and strength.

Set the tone for a supportive and informative guide for parents and caregivers.

Parents and other carers need a complete and caring guide as they start the difficult road of helping a loved one with a chronic sickness. We set the tone for a helpful and educational discussion in this chapter by stressing how important parents and other carers are to the health of the affected person and the whole family.

Empathy as the Bottom Line

The main idea behind this book is that empathy is the key to providing good help. It is imperative to understand the mental ups and downs that families may go through when someone in their family has a chronic sickness. We want to make a place where parents and carers feel seen and understood by recognizing feelings from fear and loss to strength and hope. This kind of understanding makes it possible to create a guide that connects with the real-life struggles of people whose families have a chronic diseases.

A Full Understanding of Long-Term Illness

Taking an educated attitude is a powerful way to get through the complicated world of chronic sickness. The goal of this guide is to help parents and other carers fully understand the situation their loved one is experiencing. We give carers the tools to be health advocates for their families by clarifying medical terms and giving them up-to-date knowledge. This area is a reliable source of information that offers parents and carers the tools they need to make intelligent choices and find their way around the healthcare system.

Making communication plans fit the situation

A crucial part of helping a loved one with a chronic illness is being able to talk to them. This chapter discusses customized ways to talk to people, focusing on the importance of age-appropriate conversations with kids and honest, open discussions within the family. We detail how to create a space where people feel comfortable asking questions, having their worries heard, and expressing their feelings. This guide aims to give parents and other carers the tools they need to have difficult talks sensitively and clearly by giving them helpful communication tips.

Making decisions together

The road through a chronic illness is a group effort. Parents and other carers are not the only ones who have to make decisions and care for kids. This part of the guide talks about how to build a joint family unit by getting everyone involved in talking about care plans, changes to the family's lifestyle, and mental support. Families can make their support system better and more flexible by encouraging everyone to take responsibility for their part. This way, the support system can change as the needs of the loved one change.

Putting together a support system

This guide stresses how important it is to build a network of friends, family, and neighborhood tools because it knows how important it is to have outside support. We talk about fundamental ways to reach out to others, teach them about the problems people face, and build a support network beyond the close family. We want to reinforce the idea that no one should deal with the challenges of a chronic sickness alone by advising on how to get professional help, like support groups or counseling.

Taking Care of the Well-Being of Carers

It can be hard on your mind and body to take care of a loved one who has a long-term sickness. This part stresses the importance of putting the carer's well-being first. This guide aims to keep carers from burnout by giving them valuable self-care tips, dealing with stress, and getting a break. It emphasizes that the carer's health is directly connected to the family's health, calling for a more complete approach to help.

Teaching kids to be resilient

Children need extra help and care because they are more likely to be affected emotionally by long-term sickness. This part of the guide talks about how to help kids become more resilient while considering their needs and reactions. Parents and carers can make it easier for kids to deal with the problems that come up because of a loved one's long-term illness by giving them age-appropriate ways to cope, advice on how to talk about their worries, and a safe place to be.

Promoting a Positive View of Things

Keeping an upbeat attitude can help you deal with the problems that come with having a chronic sickness. This book tells parents and other adults who care for kids to enjoy small wins, be thankful, and remember the happy times. By changing their focus from only seeing problems to seeing hope and strength, families can create a positive setting for everyone.

A Place to Get Ongoing Help

As we wrap up this chapter, we want to stress that this guide is not a one-time fix but a permanent source of help. Parents and carers can refer back to this guide for ideas, support, and ideas as the journey through a chronic sickness goes on. As families' needs change, it adapts to them and gives them the tools they need to build an intense, helpful, and well-informed atmosphere.

Chapter 2: Understanding Children's Perspectives

Explore how children perceive illness of a loved one.

When looking at the complex web of a family with a chronic illness, it is essential to remember the vital but often ignored part: how children understand and deal with the problems caused by a loved one's sickness. Through the lens of illness, this chapter looks into the rich and varied landscape of children's perspectives. It breaks down their emotional reactions and gives parents and carers the tools to help their kids through this difficult journey.

The Truth of Understanding

Children look at illness differently because they are naturally curious and emotional. This part talks about how kids can try to understand by asking questions that show how naturally curious they are. It's important to recognize and encourage this interest to promote open conversation and create a safe space for kids to share their thoughts and feelings.

How it affects kids' emotions

An illness that lasts for a long time can affect a child's emotions and make them feel a range of emotions that may be hard to explain. As they deal with the changes in their family, they may feel fear, confusion, sadness, or even guilt. This part of the chapter discusses the mental effects on kids, showing how hard it is for them to find their way in these unknown waters. Parents and other adults caring for kids can ensure they get the support and encouragement they need by knowing these feelings.

Talking to People of the Right Age

Knowing that kids of different ages have different levels of cognitive understanding makes it very important to adjust how you talk to them to fit their needs. In this part, we'll talk about how to speak to a child about a loved one's long-term illness in a way appropriate for their age and level of growth. The goal is to ensure all children feel educated and involved in the family story. This can be done through simple answers for younger children and more in-depth talks with teenagers.

How Siblings Play a Part

When a family has more than one child, a chronic illness affects more than just the person who has it. It also affects relatives. In this part of the chapter, the different points of view of siblings are looked at, along with the range of feelings they might feel. It shows how important it is for brothers to have a good relationship with each other, talk to each other openly, and be given the tools they need to handle their feelings. To keep the family together, it's crucial to understand how the ties between siblings work.

Ways of Coping and Being Strong

Kids and adults learn to deal with difficult situations by developing coping strategies. This part talks about how kids can deal with a loved one's long-term illness, such as finding comfort in habits and expressing themselves through art. Furthermore, the chapter explores children's natural resilience, stressing how important it is to recognize and support this resilience as an essential part of their emotional health.

Dealing with Fears and Misconceptions

Kids may get the wrong ideas and fears about getting sick in their made-up worlds. This part of the chapter discusses common misunderstandings kids may have and how to speak to them sensitively. Parents and other adults who care for children can help ease their fears by creating an atmosphere where questions are welcome, and misunderstandings are gently cleared up. By giving them accurate information, these people can help them form a more realistic view of the situation.

How Understanding Changes Over Time

As kids age, they learn more about how complicated long-term illnesses can be. This part talks about how a child's understanding changes over time, considering that their viewpoints will also change. It stresses how important it is to have ongoing, proper talks for the child's age. This way, parents and other adults caring for the child can stay aware of how their needs and questions change as they grow. Families can keep the conversation going and help their kids at every stage of their growth by changing the way they talk to each other.

Building compassion and empathy

Children can learn to care about others and understand how they feel when a loved one has a long-term illness. This part talks about how parents and other adults who care for kids can encourage these traits, focusing on how important it is to teach kids to be understanding, helpful, and not judgemental. Families can create an environment where kids not only understand the difficulties of having a long-term sickness but also actively add to a culture of care and support within the family by teaching empathy from a young age.

Getting help from a professional

To wrap up this chapter, it's important to remember that it might take professional help to understand how kids feel about a loved one's long-term sickness. Child experts, counselors, or support groups that focus on kids' needs can help you understand and deal with the unique problems kids may face. This part stresses how important it is to get help from outside sources to add to the work of parents and carers. This way, kids with chronic illnesses can ultimately be helped more.

Common fears, misconceptions, and concerns children may have

When a loved one has a long-term illness, children often have a lot of fears, misconceptions, and worries because they are still young and haven't lived much. Parents and other adults caring for kids need to understand these worries to help and talk about these problems with understanding and clarity. Here, we talk about some fears, misunderstandings, and concerns that kids may have:

1. Being wary of what you don't know

Kids may fear the unknown, which is one of their main fears. People with chronic illnesses often face uncertainty, changes in their habits, and possible changes in how their families interact. Kids may be afraid of the unknown, which can make them worry about what the future holds. Giving kids regular information, sticking to routines when you can, and letting them know they can always ask questions to understand better what's going on are all ways to deal with this fear.

2. False beliefs about getting the illness

Kids, particularly younger kids, may have wrong ideas about how diseases spread. They might be afraid that they will "catch" the long-term illness from a family member or friend who already has it. It's essential to clarify that many chronic diseases are not infectious and can't be passed on through everyday encounters. Giving age-appropriate answers about the illness can clear up these misunderstandings and stop people from worrying for no reason.

3. Fears for the loved one's health and safety

Children may worry about the health of a loved one affected because they think that person is in pain or trouble all the time. To ease these worries, it's crucial to have open and age-appropriate conversations about the illness, how it's being treated, and the medical care being given. Children may feel less worried if they know that the person who is sick has a healthcare team trying to ensure they are healthy.

4. Worry about how family roles will change

Family jobs and tasks often change when someone has a long-term illness. Children might be afraid that their part or other family members' roles will change, making them feel less stable. Talking openly about these changes, reassuring kids that they will still be loved and supported by their families, and giving them age-appropriate tasks can all help reduce the stress of changes in family relationships.

5. Worries about being a bother

Some kids who feel very responsible may worry that they are too much for their family. They might be afraid that their wants or worries will make things even more stressful than they already are. It's important to stress that family members should be encouraged to talk about feelings and ask for help. This worry can be eased by recognizing their part and letting them know they are not a bother.

6. Wrong ideas about what caused the illness

Kids might get wrong ideas about what caused the long-term illness, thinking it was something they did or didn't do. It is imperative to get rid of any feelings of blame or guilt and give accurate information about where the illness came from. This keeps kids from feeling responsible for things they don't need to be and creates a safe space where they can learn that illnesses aren't their fault.

7. The fear of losing a loved one who is sick

When a child has a loved one with a long-term illness, they often worry about losing them. They might be afraid that they will lose the ill family member, either because of how bad the illness is or because of false beliefs about how chronic conditions work. Children can feel less scared if they are reassured and given age-appropriate information about the treatment plan and outlook. This will help them understand what is going on better.

8. Worries about relationships with other people

Children may worry about how their friends or family will see them or a loved one who is sick. A significant stress source is the fear of being judged or looked down upon by friends and classmates. Kids can feel more confident in their social relationships if they talk openly about building a support network, teaching friends about the sickness, and teaching sensitivity.

9. Stress about their health

Kids can get worried about their health sometimes, especially if they have a chronic illness that runs in their family. To ease these worries, you should give them correct information about the genetic aspects of the disease, if relevant, and stress the significance of regular check-ups and healthy habits to keep them healthy.

10. Fears about how it will affect daily life

Kids may be worried about how the long-term illness will affect their daily lives, such as their ability to do leisure activities or go on family trips. To deal with these worries, you must find a balance between keeping things normal and getting used to the changes the illness requires. Kids can feel more in charge of their daily lives when they are involved in talks about changes and the search for creative solutions.

Insights into tailoring conversations based on different age groups with examples.

It's essential to ensure that conversations about a loved one's chronic sickness are tailored to each age group so that the information given is suitable, easy to understand, and helpful. With examples, here are some ideas on how to start a talk with kids of different ages:

1. **Kids in preschool (ages 2 to 5):**

An idea: It can be hard for pre-schoolers to understand vague ideas. Often a simple and straightforward explanation and pictures can help them understand.

Example of a Conversation Parent: "You know how when we have a cold, we need to rest to feel better? That's like something my grandmother has, but it lasts longer. You can't catch it; the doctors are ready to help her improve. Why don't we make her feel better by drawing her pictures together!"

2. **Early childhood (ages 6 to 10):**

An idea: This age group of kids is more interested and is learning more about how things work and what causes what. Some people worry about how the sickness will impact or change their daily lives.

Example of a Conversation Parent: "You know that different parts of our bodies work together, right?" Well, sometimes, one part needs extra care to stay healthy. This is what's going on with Aunt Sarah. We may need to make changes, but we're all working together to ensure she knows she is loved and cared for.

3. **Tweens (11–13 years old):**

An idea: Tweens understand the world more deeply and may be aware of how the illness affects how their family works. They might have more detailed questions about how to treat it and what the outlook is.

Example of a Conversation Parent: "You're getting old enough to know more about health now." Your uncle is quite ill but he has a group of doctors helping him deal with it. There may be changes, but we're all getting used to them. We can look things up together or talk to the doctor as a family if you have questions.

4. **Teenagers (14–18 years old):**

An idea: Teenagers want more freedom and may be worried about how the long-term sickness will affect their plans for the future and the mental health of a loved one who is involved.

Example of a Conversation Parent: "I like that you're becoming more independent. We're caring for your sister's health together, but I want you to know what you need to know. We can talk about the treatment plan together, and if you are worried or have questions about the future, we can do that, too. "How you feel is important, and this is a family matter."

Tips for Customising Conversations in General:

1. Use Age-Appropriate Language: Make sure the child understands by changing your words and phrases based on their growth stage.

2. Tell kids it's okay to ask questions: Involving them in the talk makes them feel important.

3. Assure the children they are loved and that the family works together to help the sick person.

4. Tell the truth but stay positive: Tell the truth, but put it in a good light when you do so. Bring up the support system and the steps that are being taken to handle the issue.

5. Use metaphors and analogies: Use of analogies or metaphors can help people understand complicated ideas better. For instance, you could say that the body is like a team and that sometimes one person needs extra help.

6. Adapt as Needed: Watch how the child responds and change how you talk to them based on what you see. Some people might want more information, some less, and others might need more time to think before they ask.

Talking to kids appropriately for their age helps make the home a safe place where kids can feel heard, understood, and involved in the family's journey through a loved one's long-term sickness.

Chapter 3: Creating an Open Dialogue

The importance of establishing an open and honest communication channel.

Setting up and keeping up an open and honest line of communication within the family is very important as you deal with a loved one's long-term sickness. This chapter talks about how important it is to have open and honest conversations, showing how these types of lines of communication can help with understanding, mental support, and strength. By stressing how important it is to talk to each other, we make it easier for families to deal with the difficulties of a chronic sickness as a group.

The Bedrock of Trust

Trust is the most essential thing in an open conversation. When a loved one has a long-term illness, trust becomes a valuable asset that strengthens family ties. When family members feel safe talking about their feelings, fears, and doubts, they are more likely to communicate openly. This trust works as a stabilizing force, bringing the family together and giving everyone a sense of shared duty as they face the challenges ahead.

Giving People Power Through Information

Open communication helps spread information, giving the family more power regarding long-term sickness. Families who know more about the condition, treatment choices, and changes that need to be made to their lifestyle are better able to handle the complicated situation. Parents and other adults who care for children can give them a sense of understanding by sharing information freely. This removes the mystery from the unknown and clears up any misunderstandings that could cause worry.

Making an Ecosystem That Works

Open conversation creates an environment where everyone in the family can help each other. It lets people express their feelings, worries, and weaknesses without fear of judgment. Children are more likely to be able to handle the mental challenges that come with a loved one having a long-term illness if they feel heard and understood. This setting of support becomes a stronghold that improves mental health and lets family members lean on each other for emotional support.

How to Have Conversations with People of Different Ages

Knowing that family members are of different ages means that talks must be tailored to each person. Here are some ideas for how to have discussions with kids of different ages, along with examples of how parents and other adults can do it:

1. Kids in preschool (ages 3 to 5): Pre-schoolers are naturally interested and easily swayed, and they learn best through hands-on experiences. Talk about the illness and use pictures or books for the child's age to help them understand.

For example, "[Loved One] is sick, just like our bodies get sick every once in a while." We're all here to help and love them because that means they need extra care.

2. Kids in school (ages 6 to 12): Kids in school can understand more complicated ideas but may still be sensitive to changes. Asking questions and giving honest, age-appropriate answers will help kids feel like they are part of the process and that you understand them. **In this case:** "[Loved One] has a condition that needs ongoing care." We might have to make some changes, but we'll figure it out as a team. Do you need help with something?"

3. Teenagers (13–18 years old): Teenagers want to be independent and may have a better grasp of what's happening. Please include them in conversations about how the illness affects their daily lives. This will allow them to voice their worries and give you information about the bigger picture. "I want you to know what's going on with

[Loved One]'s health," for example. It could change our schedules, and I'm here to discuss how we can handle things together. What do you think about this?"

4. Young adults and up: The conversation should shift towards making decisions together for older family members. Give them specific information about their treatment plans and include them in discussions about long-term issues. Respect their right to privacy while building a sense of shared responsibility. "Because of the nature of [Loved One's] illness, we must make some important choices." I value your opinion, and we must talk about how we can help each other and [Loved One] through this. What do you think our family's role should be?"

Dealing with Emotional Responses

Open communication helps families deal with a wide range of emotional reactions. It's important to recognize and talk about your feelings, from shock, anger and fear to hope and strength, to keep your mental balance. The conversation becomes a therapeutic place where people can find comfort and support by talking about feelings freely and confirming each family member's feelings.

Being sensitive when having challenging conversations

When someone has a chronic sickness, they will have to

have hard talks. These could include talks about how the illness worsens, possible problems, or end-of-life issues. When there is open communication, these kinds of talks can be had with care and respect. When handled with care, tough conversations can improve family bonds by creating a space for shared grief, understanding, and decision-making.

Getting help from a professional

Even though direct communication is beneficial, there may be times when you need to get help from a professional. Therapists, counselors, or support groups for people with chronic illnesses can help families communicate better by giving them helpful information and suggestions. Recognizing that communication can be challenging and being willing to get help from outside sources shows that the family is committed to maintaining a healthy conversation.

Maintaining the Open Line of Communication

To wrap up this chapter, it's important to remember that keeping the lines of communication open is an ongoing process. As someone with a chronic illness goes through changes, so should the way they talk to their family. Family check-ins, regular family talks, and time for each person to speak out all help to keep the lines of communication open and honest. Families can deal with the challenges of a chronic illness with strength, understanding, and resolve if they create a setting where everyone's voice is heard.

Strategies for creating a safe space for children to express their feelings

For kids' mental health, it's essential to give them a safe place to talk about how they feel about a loved one's long-term illness. Giving kids a place to feel heard, understood, and encouraged makes them more resiliant and better able to handle the challenging situations they face. To make this kind of safe space, try these things:

1. **Communicating openly and honestly:** Keep the lines of communication open by telling kids they can talk or ask questions at any time. When you explain the illness, be direct and use age-appropriate language. Also, make sure they understand it correctly.

2. **Active Listening:** Pay full attention when kids talk about their feelings to practice functional hearing. Use body language, like nods, to show that you are paying attention and interested in what they are saying.

3. **Validate Emotions:** Let kids know that feeling a range of emotions is okay and even expected. Don't ignore or play down their feelings; instead, show

that you understand and care. Let them know that you also have similar feelings.

4. **Please schedule a regular time to check in:** Make it a habit to check in with them regularly and ask how they feel. This pattern gives them a set time to talk, which makes it less likely that their feelings will be bottled up.

5. **Use art and creativity:** Encourage people to share their feelings through art, drawings, or writing in a journal. Kids may find it easier to talk about their feelings through these contact forms than words.

6. **Give reassurance:** Let kids know that their feelings are okay and that having a range of emotions is normal. Tell them that talking about how they feel is an excellent way to deal with things and that they are not alone.

7. **Make a Non-Judgmental Space:** Make sure they feel safe enough to be exposed by making a space where their feelings won't be judged. Remind them that there is no "right" or "wrong" way to feel and that all their thoughts are okay.

8. **Show Emotional Expression:** Show healthy emotional expression by discussing your thoughts and feelings about the situation. This shows kids that showing their feelings is okay, which makes them feel more at ease when they do the same.

9. **Use Age-Appropriate Language:** Make sure your child can understand and participate in the chat by using language appropriate for their age and stage of growth. Don't use medical jargon or other hard-to-understand words that could confuse or overwhelm them.

10. **Involve Them in Making Decisions:** Let kids help decide how to care for a sick family member or change the family's age-appropriate everyday schedule. Being involved gives people a sense of control and power, which makes them feel safer.

11. **Support System:** Remind them that they have family members who care about them and see them as a source of support. Help them find other people who will support them, like teachers or friends, whom they can talk to if needed.

12. **Professional Support:** You might want help from a child psychologist or counselor, especially if you see signs of long-term distress or mental health problems. With the help of professional advice, kids can learn specific ways to deal with their thoughts.

13. **Celebrate Positive Communication:** Let them know you appreciate it when they talk about their feelings. Feedback helps people feel more comfortable talking and builds trust in the communication process.

14. **Be patient and open to change:** Keep in mind that kids may need time to work through their feelings, which may change as they age. Be open to changing your plans based on how they understand and what they need from you.

Examples of age-appropriate language and explanations.

Kids in preschool (ages 3 to 5): Using easy words and clear explanations when talking to pre-schoolers about a loved one's long-term illness is essential. You could say, "Our bodies get sick sometimes, and that's what's happening with [Loved One]." Like when you have a cold, they need extra help and care. They can count on our help and love, just like when you are sick.

Kids in school (ages 6 to 12): For kids in school, you can give them more in-depth but still simple answers. "You know how different parts of our bodies work together? And yes, one part can get sick every once in a while. That's what's happening with [Loved One]. The doctors are helping and we're all here to help and look after them. We can talk about your thoughts and feelings if you want to.

Teenagers (13–18 years old): When talking to teens, it's essential to recognize that they are learning more and include them in conversations. "Please ensure you know what's happening with [Loved One]'s health. Their body has some problems, but it's a bit complicated. We get care from the doctors, and our family works together to help them. I care about your thoughts and want to know your feelings about everything. "We're a team, and what you say matters."

Young Adults and Up When talking to older family members, it can get easier to work together. Because of how sick [Loved One] is, important choices must be made. I believe our family must talk about this. Your thoughts and points of view are essential. Let's discuss how we can help [Loved One] and each other get through this. What do you think our roles should be? Do you have any ideas on how to help?"

Using Language That Is Right for Your Age: No matter what age, it's essential to use language that is right for that age and avoid medical jargon and other complicated words. For children, you could say, "Their body has not felt well for a long time" instead of "They have a chronic condition." You can add more medical terms for teenagers and describe them as needed. "The doctors diagnosed [Loved One] with a chronic illness, which means they need ongoing care and attention."

Dealing with Concerns: Having someone listen is essential for people of all ages. You could say, "I understand if this seems strange or scary. You can feel that way. We can talk about it and work through any worries you have. What are you thinking about?" Kids feel encouraged and given a safe place to talk about their fears when asked questions.

Rest assured: Speaking openly and listening actively is vital. "We are all here for each other, even though [Loved One] has some health problems. We immensely love and care about you and work through things together. You're not the only one going through this, and it's okay to feel different things. We'll be together through everything because we're a family. "

Putting together a unified story: Telling a suitable tale is essential regardless of age. "This is something our whole family is going through together. We will figure out what to do about [Loved One's] disease together and be there for each other every step of the way. We're strong enough to handle this as a team because it's part of our journey.

Chapter 4: Addressing Emotional Responses

The emotional impact a loved one's chronic illness can have on children.

When a loved one has a long-term illness, it affects children in ways that go beyond their physical health. It changes how they feel about the world and how they understand it. In this chapter, we'll start to look at the complicated feelings kids may have when they learn that a family member has a long-term illness. By putting light on these complex emotional issues, we hope to give parents and carers new ideas and ways to deal with the problems, creating an atmosphere of understanding, support, knowledge, love and strength.

The First Shock and Confusion

When a loved one's long-term illness is revealed, it usually sets off a wave of emotions, with shock and confusion being the first feelings that come to mind. This can be very scary for kids because they must deal with the quick changes in their everyday lives. Families may question what the sickness is, what it means, and how it affects their daily lives. To deal with this initial shock, parents and children need to talk openly, give children knowledge that is right for their age, and reassure them that it is expected to feel confused.

Worry and fear

Fear and worry often go along with the unknown that comes with having a chronic sickness. Children may fear the unknown, worry about the well-being of the loved one who is affected, or worry about how things might change in the family. Recognising and talking about these fears is essential as well as giving comfort and information to help ease worry. Giving kids a place to discuss their concerns without fear of judgment builds trust and a sense of safety.

Sadness and Loss

A chronic illness adds a sense of loss and grief to the family dynamic. Children may be sad about what they see as the loss of routine, the possibility of changes in their relationship with a loved one who has been affected, or the realization that life may not go as planned. To get through these feelings, it's crucial to validate the grieving process, let kids know it's okay to be sad about the changes and create an atmosphere where they feel safe talking about their sadness.

Sadness and Pain

Because chronic illnesses last for a long time, they can make kids feel sad and hurt all the time. It can be hard on your emotions to see a loved one fight, whether it's physically or mentally. To recognize and deal with these feelings, you can give kids chances to talk about them, give them ways to express themselves, and reassure them that being sad is a normal reaction to a challenging situation.

Feeling guilty and blaming yourself

Children often take what happened to their loved one personally and feel guilty or blame themselves. They might think that they made the sick family member sick or that their actions made things more challenging for the ill family member. It is vital to clear up these misunderstandings and reassure them that the illness is not their fault and that they are not to blame for what is happening. To deal with feelings of sorrow, it's essential to talk about them openly and clear up any confusion.

Getting mad and upset

When kids deal with the effects of a long-term illness on their lives, they may feel angry and frustrated (and in turn guilty for feeling this way). They might think things aren't fair, be angry at the situation, or be upset that they can't change anything. Valuing these feelings and giving people healthy ways to share them is very important. Helping kids talk about their anger and rage can help them find ways to deal with them and better understand their emotional world.

How it affects siblings' emotions

As they deal with the difficulties of a loved one's chronic illness, siblings may feel remarkably different feelings. Anger, jealousy, or being ignored may surface as the focus moves to the affected family member. To deal with these feelings, siblings need to talk to each other freely, recognize their emotions, and have chances to share experiences and get help.

The effect on schoolwork and social relationships

A child's mental burden from a loved one's long-term illness can spread to other areas of their life, hurting their schoolwork and relationships with other kids. Kids may find it hard to focus, change their behavior, or pull away from social activities. Finding these effects early on and working with teachers, school counselors, and friends can help build a network of support that looks out for the child's overall health.

Ways of Coping and Being Strong

Kids and adults learn to deal with difficult situations by developing coping strategies. It's important to recognise and support these ways of living to build resilience. Doing things they enjoy, allowing open conversation, and giving them ways to express themselves all help them learn healthy ways to deal with stress. Focusing on the strengths and perseverance that are already present in every child can help them handle the mental challenges that come with a loved one's long-term illness.

Why it's Important to Get Help from Outside Sources

To wrap up this look at emotional reactions, it's important to stress how important it is to get help from Professional help from therapists, counselors, or support groups that focus on the needs of children and can give you valuable ideas and tactics. Giving kids more ways to get help reinforces the notion that they are not alone in dealing with these mental problems and that help is available when they need it.

Guidance on supporting children through grief, fear, and uncertainty.

A sensitive and caring method is needed to help children deal with sadness, fear, and uncertainty when a loved one has a long-term illness. Grief, fear, and doubt are complicated feelings that show up differently for each child. Parents and other adults who care for children can help them deal with these challenging feelings safely and firmly by advising them on their needs.

1. Communicate openly and honestly: Set up a way to talk that is open and honest to start. Help the kids talk about how they feel and think about the illness. Please talk about the situation in a way that is appropriate for their age and be honest about their questions and worries. Tell them it's okay to have a lot of different feelings and that you're here to listen and help them.

2. **Their feelings are real:** Accept that kids are sad, scared, or unsure, and tell them that these are normal reactions to a challenging situation. Don't brush off or downplay their feelings; show that you understand and care. Tell them it's okay to be sad, scared, or unsure.

3. **Make a place where people feel safe expressing themselves:** Give kids a place or a regular time to talk about their feelings without fear of being judged. Let them know that you understand and value how they feel. Let kids express themselves in ways that feel normal by giving them creative tools like drawing, writing in a journal, singing songs, or telling stories.

4. **Make the process of grieving normal:** Help kids understand that it's okay to feel sad when you lose someone and that it can look different. Tell them that it's okay if their feelings change as time goes on because grief is a process. Talk about or show how

others have dealt with similar situations and stress that everyone handles loss uniquely.

5. **Give Age-Appropriate Information:** Make sure the information you give the child about the illness fits with their age and level of growth. Don't give them too many complicated details; give them enough to understand what's happening. When they ask you a question, be honest. If you don't know the answer, tell them you'll look it up together.

6. **Keep things stable and on a routine:** Make sure the child's daily life stays steady and on a routine as possible. When dealing with the unknowns that come with a loved one's long-term illness, predictability can be a comfortable base. Ensure their plan has things that don't change, like meal times, bedtimes, and school events.

7. **Try to get in touch with the affected loved one:** Help the child and the involved loved one have proper relationships for their age. This can mean doing things the kid likes, spending quality time together, or telling stories. Please encourage them to talk to each other freely, building a bond that lets the child say what they're feeling and ask questions directly.

8. **Deal with fears and doubts:** Talk to the child about their fears and doubts about the future. Assure them by explaining what is being done to deal with the illness and stressing the help available in the family.

Use real-life examples to show what is being done, like going to the doctor, making a treatment plan, or getting help from family and friends.

9. **Include Them in Decision-Making (If Appropriate):** If it's okay, include children in decision-making about how to care for a loved one who is sick. This can consist of talking about changes to daily routines and family duties or even, if they are old enough, taking part in talks about their health care. Their participation can give them a sense of control and belonging in how the family deals with long-term sickness.

10. **Get professional help:** Know when you need professional help. Child psychologists, counselors, or support groups focusing on kids' needs can help kids deal with sadness, fear, and confusion by giving them specific advice and tools. It's not a sign of weakness to get professional help. Instead, it's a proactive step towards providing the child with the best tools for mental health.

11. **Encourage Peer Support:** Help people connect with others who may have been through similar things. This can be especially helpful for older kids and teens, who may feel better talking about their problems with people who understand. Encourage making friends and talking to classmates or friends who can help you in other ways.

12. **Show examples of healthy ways to deal with stress:** Show that you have healthy ways of coping by taking care of your feelings healthily. Many times, kids learn by watching how people act around them. Talk about the nutritional and helpful ways you deal with stress, worry, or sadness, like working out, doing artistic things, or asking friends for help.

13. **Celebrate small wins and ways to deal with stress:** Celebrate the child's small successes and how they deal with stress. Recognizing good behavior helps people do more, whether talking about their feelings, trying something new, or just getting through a tough day. Celebrate the child's strength and resilience, giving them confidence when things go wrong.

14. **Review your communication with the child again and make changes as needed.** Know that the child's mental needs may change over time. Talk to them about the illness repeatedly, and ask how they're feeling, what they understand, and if they have any worries. I am willing to change how you talk to them based on their feelings and let them know you're open to talking to them again.

Age-appropriate coping mechanisms for emotional well-being.

Kids in preschool (ages 3 to 5): Nonverbal coping methods benefit pre-schoolers because they often can't explain their feelings with words. Imaginary play, drawing, coloring, and other creative activities can help people feel better. Routines and tasks you do daily give you a sense of security. Also, showing how you feel through your body, like hugging a favorite stuffed animal, can help. For toddlers, comfort and routine are essential parts of age-appropriate ways to deal with stress that help them handle their feelings in a way that fits with their level of development.

Teenagers in school (ages 6 to 12): Kids get a better handle on their feelings and can use a more significant range of ways to deal with them. Promoting open conversation is vital so that talking about feelings is easier. Journaling or having a diary is a way to cope. Activities like sports, yoga, or just playing outside can help you reduce worry and pent-up energy. Books and other tools that are right for their age can be used to help them understand and deal with their feelings. Also, promoting social ties, like those with friends, family, or a support group, can help people deal with their emotions and offer support.

Teenagers (13–18 years old): Teenagers are dealing with complicated feelings and becoming more aware of their own mental health. Writing in a journal is still helpful because it gives you a private place to think about yourself and your feelings. Awareness and relaxation techniques, like meditation or deep breathing exercises, can help you deal with stress. Encouraging artistic activities like art, music, and writing lets people express their feelings. Teenagers must have a good mix of school, leisure activities, and free time. It's getting more and more critical for people who are dealing with the mental challenges of a loved one's chronic illness to get help from other people or professional   counseling.

Young Adults and Up Family members who are older, young adults and beyond, may find comfort in a mix of coping techniques that meet their changing needs. Regular physical activity, whether by yourself or with a group, is good for your health. It's essential to keep up a robust support system of friends, family, and maybe even support groups with people who are going through similar problems. Mindfulness practices, like guided images or meditation, can help you deal with stress. Going to counseling or therapy with a professional gives you a safe place to talk about your feelings and ways of marketing. People in this group can decide how to care for and support a loved one who is sick or injured, and as they get older, they gain more independence. This gives them a sense of control and agency.

Coping Strategies That Work for Everyone: There are some ways to deal with stress that work for everyone, no matter what age. Setting up a pattern gives you order and a sense of predictability, which can help you deal with uncertainty. Promoting good habits like getting enough sleep, eating well, and exercising positively affects the mental health of people of all ages. Having a good attitude is helped by doing things that make you happy and calm down, like sports, spending time in nature, or watching movies. Lastly, stressing how important it is to get help when needed, whether from family, friends, or mental health workers, encourages the idea that coping is a group effort and help is easy to find. As people get older, their ways of coping with their emotions change to reflect their growth stages and make them more self-aware. As people get older, the toolkit gets more prominent and includes more techniques. For toddlers, it has creative outlets and physical activities. For teens, it has journaling, mindfulness, and group support. Recognizing that each family member has different needs and encouraging a variety of ways to deal with stress can help build a solid and caring family unit when a loved one has a chronic illness. Giving people of different ages emotional health tools makes it easier for them to deal with their feelings in a way that makes them feel in control.

Chapter 5: Explaining the Diagnosis Together

The importance of involving children in discussions about chronic illness.

Getting kids involved in talking about the news becomes an essential part of how a family deals with a loved one's long-term sickness. This chapter details how important it is to include children in talks about chronic illness, stressing the significance of openness, education, and social support. Families can build understanding, resilience, and a power that goes beyond the challenges the sickness brings by discussing the details of the diagnosis together.

Setting up a culture of open communication: Open communication and honesty are the building blocks of including kids in conversations about a long-term sickness. Giving kids information about the diagnosis, treatment plan, and possible problems makes it easier for them to ask questions and discuss their worries. This open culture makes kids feel valued, loved, and essential to the family. It also encourages a sense of shared duty and understanding.

How to Grow Empathy and Understanding: Kids can better understand what's happening when they are involved in conversations about long-term sickness. Parents and other adults who care for children can help them understand how complicated the illness is by giving them information appropriate for their age about the diagnosis, what it means, and the treatment plan. By spending time with and building an understanding, kids can feel empathy for their loved ones who are going through hard times. This helps build a caring and loving home environment.

Education That Is Right for Their Age: When explaining the diagnosis to a kid, it is imperative to ensure that the information is appropriate for their age and stage of growth. For younger kids, clear, simple answers that use everyday ideas can help them understand. Older kids and teens might understand the medical side of the condition better if they have more thorough information. By teaching their kids in a way that is right for their age, parents make sure that they learn what they need to know without getting too many complicated details.

Building a sense of control and freedom: Knowing the diagnosis gives kids power and freedom when they don't know what to do. Children can share their thoughts and feelings by being involved in talks about the treatment plan, lifestyle changes, and possible habits. This participation encourages the family to work together, making choices as a group, reinforcing the idea that everyone has a part to play in helping the loved one who is hurt.

Getting rid of fears and false beliefs: If kids aren't told about the ongoing illness, they might get wrong ideas and fears about it. Children have very active imaginations, they can come up with many false narratives about what is going on in the family that will only cause greater fear and stress. Including them in talks is an excellent way to clear up any confusion, allay fears, and remove false beliefs. Parents can ease their kids' worries and make them feel safe about knowing the illness and what it means by being honest about their fears and giving them the correct information.

Dealing with Emotional Responses: Children often feel a wide range of emotions when a loved one has a long-term illness. Children will often act out when they are frightened or stressed. Including them in conversations lets us talk about and explore these feelings. It gives kids a place to talk about their feelings, ask questions, and get the social support they need to deal with their complicated emotional world. Families can be more assertive and stick together through hard times by recognizing and discussing their feelings.

Getting people to ask questions and be interested: Children are naturally curious, and including them in conversations makes them more likely to ask questions to show interest. A healthy interest in the diagnosis can be encouraged by ensuring that questions are accepted and answered slowly and appropriately. This constant conversation helps kids keep learning and keeps them up to date as things change, which builds their ability to adapt and gives them a sense of safety.

Putting together a helpful network: Getting the kids involved in talking about long-term illness helps the family become more generous. In particular, siblings can be very helpful when giving each other mental support. Parents can help build a solid and caring family network to help the person with the chronic illness deal with the problems by sharing information freely and encouraging communication.

Making discussions fit the needs of each person: Because every child is different, it is crucial to make sure that conversations about the condition fit each child's needs. Some kids might like getting more knowledge and involvement, while others might do better with a more gradual and controlled method. By changing the way you talk to kids based on their nature and how they deal with stress, you can make sure that they understand the information in a way that is good for their mental health.

Putting the focus on the shared journey: Having kids talk about the long-term illness makes it clear that the whole family is going through the journey. The idea that everyone is in this together is strengthened by this shared understanding that brings people together and makes them more potent as a group. When families see their situation as a trip together, they build a sense of strength that helps them deal with the challenges of long-term sickness as a team.

Help and support from professionals: While it's important to include kids in talks, there are times when they could use some professional help and direction. Child experts, paediatricians, counselors, or support groups focusing on kids' needs can give you more ideas and suggestions. Professional help is constructive when dealing with complicated emotional reactions or when kids need extra help to understand the medical parts of the condition.

Creating a Culture of Strength: In the end, including kids in conversations about a family member's long-term illness builds an intense and understanding family atmosphere. Parents and carers can help their kids' emotional health by encouraging open dialogue, ensuring knowledge fits each child's needs, and discussing feelings. When families discuss the diagnosis together, they create a supportive space based on understanding, shared duty, and a strength that goes beyond the problems caused by the chronic disease. Building a resiliency in the individual and the family as a whole is an important part of journeying through stressful and difficult times.

Tools and resources for explaining medical concepts in a family-friendly way.

To talk about medical ideas with kids in a good way for the whole family, you must be careful and use tools and resources that make complicated information relevant and easy to understand. Here are some tools and resources that can help parents and other adults who care for kids with this challenging job and ensure that kids can understand medical ideas without getting too stressed or confused.

1: Children's books and telling stories: Use children's books specifically written to explain medical ideas in a way that is right for their age. Often, these books use simple words and figures that are easy to relate to and explain big ideas. Storytelling keeps kids' minds active, which makes it easier for them to understand medical words and processes they don't know.

2. Websites and apps that let you interact: Check out websites and apps that are meant to teach kids about the body, illnesses, and medical processes that are engaging. These digital tools often use games, graphics, and other dynamic features to make learning fun and interesting. Because respected healthcare groups and trainers make some platforms, you can be sure their information is correct and trustworthy.

3: Videos and animations for learning: Use teaching animations and movies that break down medical ideas. There may be feeds on sites like YouTube that are just for teaching medical topics in a way that kids can understand. Visual tools can help people understand more, especially those who learn best by seeing.

4. Medical play sets: Buy medical play sets with dolls and safe medical tools for kids. Kids can use these kits as props to act out medical situations, which helps them get better at using tools and following instructions. Medical play can help make medical ideas less scary by letting kids try and connect with them.

5. People working with children: Talk to child life specialists and trained professionals who explain medical ideas to kids. As people who work in healthcare, these experts can help kids understand their loved one's situation by suggesting age-appropriate words, tools, and activities.

6: Social Stories: Use simple words and pictures in your social stories to explain medical treatments, hospital stays, or changes in your routine. Social stories give kids an organized and predictable way to get knowledge, which makes them less anxious and helps them get ready for what to expect.

7. Picture books with your name on them: Make personalized picture books with pictures of family members and specifics about the sickness of a loved one. Personalization makes the information more beneficial for the child and lets medical ideas be explained in a way that fits their needs.

8. Charts and models of the body: Use charts and models of the human body made for kids. Using these visual tools to teach basic anatomy and how different body parts work can be constructive. Some models let kids explore and ask questions by being involved.

9. Brochures and pamphlets for kids: Look for handouts and brochures made for kids and given out by healthcare organizations. Most of the time, these tools are made to make medical ideas simple enough for kids to understand. They might discuss common diseases, medical tests, or different treatment methods.

10. Art and craft projects: Get kids involved in arts and crafts projects where they can make models of medicine ideas. For instance, they can use everyday things to make a human body model or draw pictures showing how a specific illness affects people. Hands-on tasks help kids learn and remember what they've learned.

11. Websites that help kids learn online: Check out websites made just for kids with health and physics lessons. Some platforms have games, quizzes, and live lessons that teach kids about the body and other common health subjects.

12. Family Talks and Meetings: Set up family groups where you can talk freely about medical ideas. Help kids talk about their thoughts and ask questions. During these talks, use a whiteboard or pictures to help explain things. This will make the learning process more collaborative and open to everyone.

13. People who work as pediatric health educators: Contact pediatric health trainers who explain medical information to kids. These experts can help families talk about medical ideas in a way that is sensitive to children's growth needs by giving them tools, advice, and plans.

14. Museums of Children's Health: Visit health sites or displays about the body and health of kids. Often, these educational areas have medical-themed exhibits that kids can learn about while having fun.

15. Groups that help families: Join support groups for families who are going through the same physical problems. Talking to other families about your experiences can help you understand how they have taught their kids about medical ideas. Support groups can also help you feel better and give you hope.

Finally, to teach kids medical ideas in a fun way for the whole family, you need a mix of exciting tools and resources. Adapting the method to the kid's age, hobbies, and way of learning makes these tools work better. The goal is to create a caring and helpful space where kids can feel safe and educated as they deal with the complicated issues that come up because of a loved one's illness.

Examples of collaborative approaches to understanding the diagnosis

Family members, especially children, should be involved in talks and choices about a loved one's chronic illness as part of collaborative approaches to understanding a diagnosis. These methods aim to create a space where everyone can learn, talk, and help each other. These are some examples of ways to work together:

1. Meetings with family: Set up regular meetings with your family to discuss the news. This way of working together lets everyone be there, say what they think, and ask questions. You might want to use graphs or charts to help explain medical ideas in a way that is easy for everyone to understand.

2. Collaboration in research: Get everyone in the family, even the kids, to work together to study the specific chronic sickness. This can be done by reading articles suitable for their age, watching educational videos together, and discussing what they've learned from their study. Collaborative learning brings people together and builds up their knowledge.

3. Discussions with people of different generations: Encourage conversations between grandparents, parents, and children where everyone can share their thoughts and experiences. Older family members can give you advice and background, while younger family members can give you new ideas. This conversation between generations helps everyone understand the findings better.

4. Expression through art: Encourage artistic expression as a way for everyone to work together to understand the condition. Families with a member with a chronic illness can work together on an art project that shows the journey, feelings, and problems that come with it. This group art project can be a great way to get people to talk to each other.

5. Workshops where you can interact: Set up engaging workshops or lessons that are led by people who work in healthcare. During these meetings, games and talks that are appropriate for the age of the family members can help everyone, even kids, understand medical ideas. Interactive learning keeps people interested and helps them understand the findings better.

6. Making decisions together: Set up ways for everyone in the family to help make decisions. This includes discussing possible treatments, changes to the person's lifestyle, and daily activities. Making sure everyone has a say in decisions builds a sense of togetherness and duty among everyone.

7. Making a binder with family resources: Make a family reference binder with essential people's diagnoses, care plans, and contact information. Everyone in the family should help you add this book to it. This website can be a central place where everyone can find information.

8. Writing in a family journal: Start a family log where everyone, even the kids, can write down their feelings, thoughts, and questions about the news. Sharing journal writings at family gatherings encourages open conversation and shows how each family member sees things.

9. Using technology: Use technology to help kids understand the condition. Virtual tours of medical facilities, engaging apps that teach medical ideas in a way that kids can understand, and telehealth appointments are all things that can help families learn together.

10: "Storytelling Circles": Set up storytelling circles where family members can share their stories about a long-term sickness. This way of telling stories together helps kids feel connected to the journey, making them feel like they are all part of the story and getting it.

11. Visits to people in health care: Make appointments for your family to see doctors and nurses. With this collaborative method, everyone can participate in conversations with medical workers, ask questions, and fully understand the diagnosis and treatment plan.

12. Real-Life Role-Playing Situations: Play role-playing games that reflect different parts of dealing with a chronic illness. This practice can help everyone in the family, especially kids, think about different events they might face and get ready for them.

13: Setting goals together: Set goals together as a family that spells out what you will all do to help the hurt person. This could include jobs, responsibilities, or changes to how you live that everyone agrees to work on together.

14. Check-ins regularly: Set up regular check-ins where everyone in the family, including the kids, can say what they think and feel about what's going on. This kind of contact helps deal with new issues and ensures everyone is on the same page.

15. Family Support Network: Make a support system for your family that goes beyond your close family. Work with close friends, extended family, and community tools to build a robust support system that helps the family understand and deal with things better.

Using these joint methods in the family can make it a more helpful and well-informed place. By including everyone in the family, even the kids, in learning about the diagnosis, families can face the challenges of a long-term illness together with unity, kindness, and strength.

Chapter 6: Maintaining Stability and Routine

Maintaining stability and routine for children.

In the complicated web of a family dealing with a loved one's long-term illness, keeping children's security and routines strong stands out as a critical source of support. When someone in the family has a long sickness, it can cause many problems and uncertainty, considerably affecting the children. This chapter details how vital stability and patterns are in a child's life during these times, showing how they can provide comfort, normalcy, and mental health.

The Basis of Predictability: For kids whose lives are complicated by a loved one's long-term illness, stability and habit help make things more predictable. With all the unknowns that can happen, having an organized daily routine can help you feel safe. Following a pattern, like getting up at the same time or doing the same things every day, can help kids feel more stable and confident as they deal with different feelings.

Emotional Safety: Feeling emotionally safe is essential for kids, and having a stable daily routine is a big part. Kids feel mentally safe when they know what to expect from family meals, bedtime routines, and everything everyone does together. When dealing with the problems and changes that can come with a loved one's long-term illness, this mental steadiness is even more critical. **Maintenance of Normalcy:** Routine is vital in a child's daily life. The predictability is soothing. When medical visits, treatment plans, or changes in family dynamics make life less stable, sticking to as many basic habits as possible can help you feel like things are more normal. It tells kids that even though things are hard, some things will always be the same in their lives.

A Way to Cope with Change: When a family member has a long-term illness, their jobs and tasks often change. Kids may find these changes tough to handle. Setting up and sticking to stable habits helps them deal with stress by giving them a framework for adjusting to changes in their surroundings. It helps keep things steady during change by providing security and comfort.

Encouraging Physical Health: Having regular routines helps kids stay healthy by ensuring they stick to healthy habits. Having standard food times, getting enough sleep, and having chances to be active are all essential parts of a stable routine. These things are crucial to a child's general health and can make them more robust when dealing with the mental challenges that come with a loved one's long-term illness.

Educational Continuity: Stability and habit are also crucial for school-age kids when it comes to their education. Having a regular plan for school, homework, chores, and extracurricular activities helps students feel stable and gives them a sense of continuity in their academic efforts. This security helps them learn and focus and gives them a positive way to release stress.

Feeling in charge and able to plan: When someone in the family has a long-term illness, kids may feel like they have lost power. They feel in charge and sure of their lives when they have stability and routine. For their emotional health, knowing what to expect at different times of the day gives them a structured setting where they can practice independence. If there will be a change in their plans, as much advanced notice as possible and reminders are important.

Making rituals that bring people together: Through habits, families can create traditions that bring them closer together and strengthen their relationships. Whether it's a weekly game night, a unique way to get ready for bed, or eating meals together, these habits become ways for everyone to connect. They bring happiness, fun, and time spent together, balancing the problems chronic sickness causes.

Controlling your emotions: Stability and schedule are very important for kids to keep their emotions in check. Regular schedules give people a comfortable flow that helps them feel emotionally stable. Kids can guess what will happen next, making them feel safe and allowing them to control their emotions when stressed or unsure. Gentle reminders such as "First we will see the doctor, then it will be lunchtime."

Channels of Communication: Routines make it easy for family members to talk to each other. Sharing food or going to bed at the same time every night can become time for open conversation to grow. Children can talk about their day, feelings, and thoughts in this ongoing conversation, which makes them feel heard and supported as they go through a loved one's chronic sickness or any challenging time.

To promote independence: Kids feel more independent with a stable pattern. They are more likely to take responsibility for specific tasks and duties when they know what to expect. Being independent helps them feel good about themselves and strengthens them, making it easier to deal with problems.

Be able to change your routine: Even though steadiness is essential, it's also important to know that routines need to be able to be changed when necessary. Because of how chronic illnesses work, they can bring about unexpected or immediate changes. Families can change their daily routines to make room for medical visits, treatment plans, and the loved one's changing needs. This ability to adapt ensures that security stays the same, even when things change.

Giving kids power by getting them involved: Getting kids involved in making and sticking to habits gives them power and a sense of security. Making daily plans, actions, and routines together gives everyone a sense of ownership. This shows them you respect their words, creating a cooperative and supportive family atmosphere.

Advice from professionals on routine development: In some situations, getting help from pediatric health workers or child life experts can be helpful. These professionals can give you advice on how to make habits fit the growth needs of kids, taking into account things like their age, temperament, and ways of dealing with stress. Keeping kids stable and on a routine while a loved one has a long-term illness is a method that looks at their mental, physical, and educational well-being as a whole. For kids dealing with a family member's health problems, the consistency of daily life provides comfort, strength, and a sense of connection. When families work together to set up and change habits, they create a supportive space where stability becomes a sign of normalcy and mental health amid the unknowns of a chronic disease.

Practical tips for balancing normalcy while accommodating medical needs.

In the complicated dance of dealing with a loved one's long-term illness, keeping things stable and normal becomes a vital part of helping children through the problems that come up. This chapter explores the profound importance of security and habit for children, and practical tips are given for finding a balance between normalcy and meeting medical needs. Families can provide their children a sense of safety, stability, and mental health even though their child has a chronic illness by making sure that daily life is consistent.

Why stability and routine are essential:
1. Emotional Security: Children feel emotionally safe with stability and order. People who know what to expect in their daily lives feel more stable, which can be exceptionally comforting when dealing with the unpredictability of a loved one's health.

2. Have a sense of normalcy: Keeping things stable and routine helps kids feel normal even when dealing with long-term illness. Routines, activities, and plans that are the same every day help create a comfortable environment that makes up for the changes that the medical situation has caused.

3. Ways of Dealing with Stress: Children use routine to deal with stress because it gives them a way to handle the uncertainty that come up when a family member is sick. Routines that you know give you a sense of security and control when things aren't going as planned.

4. Emotional Regulation: Routines help kids keep their emotions in check. It helps to be emotionally healthy to know what to expect and when to expect it. This is especially important when dealing with the mental highs and lows that can come with a loved one's long-term sickness.

5. Making communication easier: Having stable habits makes it easier for family members to talk to each other. Family meals or regular sleep habits make discussing problems, feelings, and new health information accessible. This makes the space safe for kids to feel heard.

6. Academic success: Stability and habit are suitable for academic success. Kids often do better when they have set daily routines like chores, study time, and hobbies outside of school. Even though things are hard at home, this consistency helps them with schoolwork.

7. Making yourself more resilient: Building grit in kids is helped by having regular habits. Being resilient means dealing with changes while keeping some sense of normalcy. This is a necessary trait when dealing with a loved one's chronic sickness.

Helpful Advice for Finding a Balance Between Normalcy and Medical Needs:

1. Make a schedule that you can change: A flexible plan that fits medical visits, treatments, and possible changes in the loved one's health is essential, even though sticking to a pattern is essential. Make sure that any changes to the plan are communicated ahead of time to avoid too many problems.

2. Put self-care first: Make sure everyone in the family, including the kids, puts self-care first. As part of this, you might set aside "quiet time" to think or do things that make you happy and calm down. Taking care of yourself is good for your mental health and strengthens you.

3. Bring kids into the planning process: Bring kids into the planning process for daily tasks and routines. If they feel like they have a say in decisions that affect their lives, it gives them power and encourages a team effort to keep things stable while meeting medical needs.

4. Set up regular routines for going to bed: Routines before bed are essential for calm. Set an average time to go to bed and do something relaxing before bed, like reading, listening to soft music, or doing relaxation techniques. Kids need to get enough good sleep for their general health.

5. Set aside time for family: Make time for family a priority in your schedule. This could be a set time for a meal, a weekly exercise the whole family does together, or a day for sharing experiences. Make time for fun! Family time makes relationships stronger and brings people closer together.

6. Talk to each other honestly: Stability depends on people being able to talk freely. Tell kids about the medical situation as much as they can handle for their age. Please encourage them to talk about how they feel and what worries them. If age appropriate, share your feelings as well. This will build trust and openness.

7. Create rituals that help you connect: Connecting practices should be a part of your daily life. These times, like a hug in the morning, a check-in in the evening, or a shared routine before a doctor's visit, bring people together and make them feel safe.

8. Organise help for schools: Make sure the child's learning needs are met by working with teachers and school officials. Share information about the long-term illness, talk about possible problems, and look into making adjustments if needed.

9. Eat well: Stability includes staying on top of your eating habits. Ensure meals are balanced and regular, and consider any health-related food limits or suggestions. Eating well is good for your health in general.

10. Plan what to do in an emergency: Keep to your routine, but be ready for emergencies with backup plans. Tell your kids about these plans, including what to do if an emergency happens out of the blue. Having clear steps in place makes things even more stable.

11. Include activities that are good for you: Add therapeutic tasks to your daily practice. This can include things like art therapy, breathing routines, or activities that take place outside that are good for your mental health. Treatments help people be more stable and resilient in general.

12. Use technology to help you out: Use technology to help with daily tasks and conversation. To remember your doctor's meetings, use apps or notes, make a shared digital calendar, or use video calls to check in with extended family members from far away.

13. Get people to help each other: Make friends with people who may be going through the same things you are.

Encourage people to make friends and talk to their teachers or friends, who can offer extra support and understanding. **14. Get help from a professional:** If you need to, talk to a counselor, therapist, or support group for help. Professionals can give you more tools and strategies to help you stay stable while meeting your medical needs and dealing with any unique mental problems that may come up.

5. Celebrate essential events and accomplishments: Family events and achievements should be recognized and celebrated. Remembering these moments, whether a good medical report, a school accomplishment, or a personal success, helps everyone feel like things are back to normal and bring everyone joy. Keeping things stable and regular is a constantly shifting balancing act that needs everyone in the family to be flexible and work together. Families can make a safe and caring space for their children where they feel linked and able to handle the challenges of a loved one's long-term illness with strength and resolve by putting stability first and meeting medical needs as needed.

Stories of families successfully navigating daily life with a loved one's chronic illness.

Getting through daily life with a loved one's chronic illness is hard, but many families have shown extraordinary strength, flexibility, and resilience in the face of hardship. These stories of people who overcame adversity inspire and teach us valuable things about keeping our lives regular while meeting medical needs.

The Thompson Family: Being Open to Change and Creativity

Taking care of a parent's long-term illness was hard for the Thompson family, who had two young children. Even though they had to go to doctor's visits and treatments, they stressed being flexible and creative to keep things feeling normal. A family schedule was made, which included both medical visits and special events. The family created a positive environment by letting the kids help plan fun activities. This turned the family's medical needs into shared experiences. Weekends became time for family trips, allowing them to get to know each other better and giving them a break from their medical obligations.

The Rodriguez Family: Making a Helpful Network

The Rodriguez family's child had a long-term illness, so friends and family who could help them became very important. They built a strong support network by getting involved with their extended family, friends, and the community. Family members took turns helping with chores around the house, friends set up carpools for medical visits, and the community came together to support the family when things got tough. Working together not only made things more accessible but also made sure that the family could keep things stable for their teen without getting too stressed out.

This is The Chen Family: Education and Empowerment.

The Chen family focused on schooling and giving their child more power because their child had a long-term sickness. They took the time to understand the physical situation fully. And in return, they taught their child about their health. The child felt in charge and understood things better through talks and learning tools that were right for their age. Together, they set up habits for taking medications and checking their health regularly. Working together gave the child power and the family a sense of responsibility and routine.

This is The Williams Family: Using Technology.

One parent in the Williams family had a long-term illness, and technology was fundamental to them. The family could stay in touch with extended family members who lived far away, thanks to virtual contact tools. Medical reports were shared on safe sites, which helped people feel more united and supported. The family also used health-tracking apps to monitor the loved one's signs and ensure everyone knew what was happening with their health. Using technology in this way became a valuable and efficient way to balance everyday life with the needs of handling long-term sickness.

The Gupta Family: Putting Self-Care and Delegation First

The Gupta family had to deal with the stresses of work, school, and a parent's long-term illness. They set up a plan that included time for leisure and personal activities because they knew how important it was to take care of themselves. In addition, they believed in the power of delegating and gave each family member specific tasks to do. By splitting up the work, they kept from getting burned out and set up a daily pattern that would last. This way of working together ensured everyone's wants and needs were met and brought the family closer.

Helpful Advice for Finding a Balance Between Normalcy and Medical Needs:

1. Make a calendar for the family: Make a shared schedule with important dates like doctor's visits, family gatherings, and fun activities. This visual guide keeps everyone on track and gives a good picture of what they must do each month.

2. Involve kids in making choices: When it's proper for their age, let kids help make decisions about long-term sickness. This can include picking out activities, making trips, or giving suggestions on how to take care of medical needs. Giving kids choices gives them a sense of control and routine.

3. Make a support system: Ask for help from family, friends, and nearby neighbors. Getting to know people who are ready to help with daily jobs or offer emotional support can make things easier and make you feel more stable.

4. Use Technology for Communication: Use technology to keep everyone updated and in touch. Family members can stay in touch even when busy, thanks to virtual communication tools, texting apps, and shared platforms allowing real-time information.

5. Teach and involve everyone in the family: Teach everyone in the family about the medical situation, ensuring the information is accessible for them to understand. Sharing information makes people more empathetic, calms them down, and ensures everyone is on the same page.

6. Make routines for every day: Do things every day as a family that bring you together. Whether it's a family meal, bedtime stories, or a morning routine, these habits give us a sense of safety and joy even when things are hard.

7. Make self-care a priority: Tell everyone in the family how important it is to care for themselves. Encourage people to do things that help them relax and feel better so that everyone has the mental and emotional strength to deal with the stresses of daily life.

8. Delegate Responsibilities: Give family members jobs and duties to do. This group effort keeps one person from getting too busy and ensures everyone does their part to keep the house running smoothly.

9. Enjoy milestones and successes: Recognise and enjoy achievements and milestones, no matter how they are. Recognizing wins in the family, whether linked to dealing with a chronic illness or personal goals, keeps everyone happy.

10. Encourage a free flow of information: Open lines of conversation so family members can talk about their thoughts, worries, and wants. A mindset of communication helps people understand each other and lets the family work together to solve problems. Families who can get through daily life with a loved one's chronic illness show how important it is to work together, be strong, and be flexible. These stories not only give hope to other families going through similar problems but also give them helpful advice. Families can find a balance between normalcy and medical needs using these tactics. This will help create a welcoming atmosphere that lives on unity and shared strength.

Chapter 7: Encouraging Empathy and Compassion

Ways to nurture empathy and compassion in children.

Fostering empathy and care in kids is a life-changing experience that does more than teach them to be kind; it changes their character. Developing understanding is especially important when a loved one has a long-term sickness. This chapter talks about ways to help kids develop these critical traits, giving them the mental tools they need to deal with illness with kindness and understanding.

1. Show others how to do it: The way people act powerfully affects children because they learn by watching. In your daily life, show others how to be attentive and caring. Kindness should be shown not only to the person with a chronic illness but also to other people. When adults give help, care about someone's well-being, or show understanding in challenging situations, kids pick up on these behaviors and make them a part of their attitudes.

2. Encourage taking a different view: Help kids learn how to see things from other people's points of view. Talk about the problems the family member with a long-term illness faces and try to picture what it would be like to be them. Have open-ended talks with your kids to help them think about how their loved one felt and what they went through. Building empathy starts with this practice, which enables you to understand how the illness affects the person more deeply.

3. Give information that is right for their age: Understanding is the first step to having empathy, and telling kids about the chronic sickness in a way that is right for their age helps them understand it better. Give them information about the medical side of the illness without giving them too much. Children can relate to their loved one's feelings more deeply and react with more understanding and kindness when they know more about them.

4. Show empathy by making chances for it: Get the kids involved in doing nice things for the family member with a long-term sickness. This could mean doing everyday jobs together, making personalized cards or pictures, or spending time together. These kinds of tasks help people understand how others feel and support the idea that small acts of kindness can significantly affect someone's health.

5. Read books and watch movies about empathy: Read books and watch movies that are about understanding, kindness, and care. Pick books and films that are proper for your child's age and show people dealing with problems, being kind, and making connections. Talk about the characters' feelings and behaviors afterward to help kids become more emotionally intelligent and empathetic.

6. Make it more accessible to show how you feel: Give the kids a safe place to talk about their feelings and worries about the long-term sickness. Please encourage them to be honest about their thoughts, whether in a talk, a drawing, or a journal. Being able to empathize with others and with their feelings grows when they are acknowledged and validated.

7. Teach people how to listen actively: You must first listen to show empathy. Kids should learn to listen actively, which means paying full attention, making eye contact, and reacting with understanding. By improving this skill, kids can better understand how their loved ones feel and what they need. This not only strengthens family ties but also makes the child more compassionate.

8. Do things that will change your point of view: Take part in tasks that help you see things from different points of view. Role-playing games can help kids understand different points of view by putting them in situations linked to chronic sickness. Kids learn to care about others by putting themselves in other people's shoes and seeing the world through their eyes.

9. Tell stories of how you've been strong: Stories about people who have been through hard times and come through them with strength and courage can be very compelling at building understanding. Tell stories about people who had long-term illnesses and show not only how hard it was for them but also how strong and determined they were to keep going. People can understand and appreciate the strength of others by reading inspiring stories.

10. Get people outside the family to do nice things: Kindness and understanding should be practiced by more than just family. Do volunteer work or acts of community service together. These activities allow kids to meet with a wider range of people going through different kinds of problems. Giving to other people's well-being builds understanding and a sense of social duty.

11. Set up a Family Empathy Jar: Put together an empathy jar where everyone in the family, even the kids, can write down kind things they did or times they felt empathy. Share these notes with your family at gatherings to honor the times when kindness was shown. The empathy jar is a physical sign of how much the family wants   to   teach   kindness.

12. Talk about your feelings openly: Encourage your family to talk about their feelings in an open way. Establish a setting where various feelings are okay, such as sadness, anger, or fear. Children learn to understand and relate to other people's emotions by recognizing and talking about their own.

13. Stress How Words Have an Effect: Consider how words can affect other people's feelings. Teach kids how important it is to be thoughtful and careful with their words, especially when talking about a long-term illness. By learning about the power of words, kids can talk to each other with understanding and respect, which makes for a more supportive and understanding family.

14. Work together on artistic expression: Do art projects with your kids that let them creatively show their understanding. Working together on art projects, like making a family empathy painting or writing a poem, helps everyone in the family share their feelings and understand each other better.

15. If you need to, get professional help: If your kids have trouble dealing with their feelings or showing understanding, you might want to get them help from a professional. Child psychologists and counselors can help kids feel better emotionally and develop knowledge by giving them methods and support designed for their needs. Furthermore, teaching kids to feel empathy and kindness when a loved one has a long-term sickness is a deep and ongoing process. When families use these tactics daily, they can make empathy a regular part of their child's personality. Developing empathy helps the child and makes it easier for the family to deal with the challenges of the child's sickness with strength, understanding, and unwavering kindness.

The role of storytelling and shared experiences in building understanding.

Sharing stories and experiences is a great way to understand each other, especially when someone you care about has a long-term sickness. Including these parts of a story helps build a shared family story, encourages understanding, and helps people understand the problems better. Let's look at what their roles are:

1. Making a collective family story: Storytelling helps make the journey of having a long-term illness into a shared family story. Families can make sense of their events together by telling stories, which create a story that ties them together. By telling this story together, we can better understand and help each other.

2. Bringing Generations Together: Storytelling brings people of different groups together by letting older family members share their knowledge and experiences with younger family members. Understanding the family's experience with chronic sickness is more accessible with this link between generations. It shows how the family has dealt with similar problems in the past.

3. Personal stories can help people understand each other better, Personal stories give people with chronic illnesses a face to the experience. Sharing personal stories about the struggles, victories, and feelings that come with the disease helps family members understand it better, which builds understanding. The person with the illness is not just a patient; through stories, they are seen as real people with a whole life.

4. **Encouraging Taking a Different View:** Stories that show shared situations help people see things from different points of view. Family members learn more about each other's feelings and thoughts, which allows them to understand how long-term illness affects everyone. This understanding of empathy is what makes family relationships strong.

5. **Open Conversation:** Storytelling makes it easier for family members to talk to each other. It gives people with chronic illnesses an organized and safe place to discuss their feelings, worries, and questions. Family members can share their experiences by telling stories and encouraging

open conversation that helps everyone understand each other better.

6. How to Handle Complicated Feelings: People with chronic illnesses often feel a lot of different emotions, and stories can help them deal with these feelings. Family members can talk about their worries, dreams, and problems through stories, which allows others to understand and help. Sharing experiences through stories helps make emotional reactions more regular, which makes the family setting more understanding and caring.

7. Learning and Dealing with Stress Together: Education through Stories: Stories can teach family members, especially children, about the medical side of a chronic illness. By adding educational parts to stories, families can remove the mystery from complicated medical ideas and help everyone understand them.

8. Coping Techniques: Stories sharing everyday situations help families discuss their problems and develop ways to deal with them. Narratives can show how people deal with problems, how resilient they are, and how their family members pull together during hard times. This shared knowledge helps the family work together better and be better prepared.

9. Bringing Attention to Resilience: Stories often show how strong people are and how they can get through hard times. Sharing stories of how people have been strong while dealing with a chronic illness makes the family more substantial. It gives the family hope, energy, and the strength to face problems as a united and determined group.

10. Building Positive Stories: Families can make positive stories about times of joy, love, and shared successes through retelling, even while remembering the hard times. These good stories help us see the family's journey more fairly, which boosts hope and a sense of belonging.

11. Creating a Sense of Community: Family stories bring people together and give them a sense of who they are. By telling stories about their experiences, family members can see they are not going on this trip alone. This shared identity creates a strong bond, supporting the idea that the family is working together to deal with the problems caused by the long-term illness.

12. Taking ownership of the story as a group: There is a sense of joint ownership over the family story when everyone shares it. Everyone tells their part of the story, changing and adding to it. Having this sense of control helps everyone understand and value the part each family member plays in the story. Finally, sharing stories and experiences is a big part of helping everyone in the family understand why a loved one has a long-term sickness. Families use stories to tell each other a shared story that shows the difficulties they faced and the strengths, courage, and understanding that made their journey a whole. Storytelling is powerful because it can bring people together through shared experiences, creating a family story that is strong, understanding, and caring.

Activities and exercises to promote a supportive family environment

It's crucial to create a caring family environment, especially when dealing with the difficulties of a loved one's long-term sickness. Family bonds can be strengthened by doing tasks and routines that help people talk to each other, understand each other, and connect. Here are some things you can do to make your family stronger:

1. Family Gatherings Setting up regular family talks will give everyone a safe place to talk. Talk about how you feel, what worries you, and any new information about the long-term illness. Encourage everyone in the family to give their opinion, which will help everyone work together and understand each other better.

2. The Gratitude Circle: Start a "gratitude circle" where everyone in the family says something they're grateful for. This helps family members realize the love and support they get from each other and keeps them in a good mood.

3. Art projects where people work together: Do art projects with other people that will help you be creative and talk to each other. Making a family painting, scrapbooking, or crafting gives everyone a chance to be artistic together, which brings people closer together.

4. Writing in a family journal: Encourage everyone in the family, even the kids, to keep journals where they can write down their feelings, thoughts, and experiences about long-term sickness. Read portions aloud at family gatherings to help everyone understand.

5. Memory Lane: Put together a "Memory Lane" by collecting family pictures, souvenirs, and other items that are important to them. Thinking about memories you have together strengthens your mental bonds and sense of belonging.

6. Supportive Message Jar: Set up a message jar where family members can write notes to each other to cheer them up, show their thanks, or show their love. If the family struggles, they can reread these words to feel better.

7. The day when roles are switched: Have a "Role Reversal Day" occasionally where family members change jobs and responsibilities. This game builds empathy by letting everyone in the family feel the problems that other family members are having.

8. Book Club for the whole family: Make a book club and choose a book or articles about chronic illnesses or coping with hard times. Talking about the topic helps everyone understand it and creates a space for honest talks.

9. Games That Help People Feel Empathy: Play games that help you understand others and work together. Family members can learn to support each other through joint board games, role-playing, and team-building activities.

10. Movie night with the family: Set aside a regular movie night with your family to watch movies or programs about people who have chronic illnesses or who have overcome adversity. After reading the stories, have a conversation to share your thoughts and feelings.

11. Shared Responsibility Board: Make a shared responsibility board where you can write down chores and duties related to long-term illness. Assign jobs to each family member and stress how important it is to work together to solve problems.

12. Letters of thanks: Get family members to write letters of thanks to each other, showing gratitude for certain traits or deeds. At family gatherings, read these letters to honor what each person has done.

13. A family cookbook: Make a family cookbook where everyone can share their favorite recipes. This group effort makes a real-world picture of shared events and shows how important it is to help each other.

14. Problems with family health: Start fitness tasks for the whole family, focusing on their physical and mental health. To support each other's health more thoroughly, this can include going for daily walks, breathing exercises, or trying new healthy foods together.

15. Get Volunteering Together: Do charity work as a family to help groups that deal with long-term illnesses or health care. Assisting other people to feel suitable supports the values of empathy, caring, and group support.

16. Come up with a coping strategy: Hold a meeting with your family to talk about ways to deal with things. Encourage everyone in the family to discuss how they deal with stress and uncertainty and share good strategies to help everyone.

17. Family Picture Board: Make a vision board for your family that shows your shared values, goals, and hopes. This action that everyone does together builds a sense of unity and purpose, reinforcing that the family is dealing with the challenges of long-term sickness as a unit.

18. Nature walks or trips: Plan trips for the whole family, like walks in nature or quiet places. Being outside helps you relax and gives your family a chance to spend time together away from the stresses of everyday life.

19. Storytelling Circle: Make a circle where family members can share personal stories, memories, or experiences. Each person should take a turn. This practice helps people get to know each other better and see things from their unique points of view.

20. Make a plan to help your family: Make a family support plan that spells out what each person can do to help the person with a chronic illness. This plan can include valuable things to do, ways to help someone feel better, and planned events for the whole family. Adding these things to your family's daily routine can help create a helpful space. The important thing is to change these ideas to fit the wants and tastes of your family. Remember that the goal is to improve relationships, encourage empathy, and encourage a sense of community as you deal with the difficulties of a loved one's long-term sickness.

Chapter no. 8: Getting kids involved in care

Families who have a loved one with a chronic sickness often work together to care for them, which can be both challenging and fulfilling. Helping and caring for kids simultaneously is a tricky mix that needs methods that are right for their age. This builds family unity and shared responsibility.

Participation Appropriate for Age:

Children at different stages of growth can understand and help care for a loved one differently. Younger kids can feel like they are contributing by doing easy things like getting a glass of water, doing light housework, or drawing happy pictures. Older children can take on more duties, like helping to remember to take medications, attending meetings with a loved one, or having deep talks about what that person needs.

1. Making a routine together: Have the kids help you make a daily schedule that includes time to care for a loved one. This could be as easy as setting aside specific times to take medications, rest, or do fun things with the other person. By taking part in making the pattern, kids learn how important order and predictability are in getting care.

2. Getting people to offer emotional support: Children can make a big difference by giving their loved ones mental support. This means paying attention to their feelings, listening carefully, and being there for them. Children can help with their physical, psychological, and emotional health by building an emotional connection with a family member.

3. Helping with daily tasks: Kids can help with different daily tasks, depending on their age and the wants of the loved one. This could mean doing light workouts together, helping to make meals, or moving around more quickly if needed. These tasks not only help out in real life, but they also bring the family closer together by letting them share experiences.

4. Taking Part in Educational Activities: Offer educational activities related to the care of the loved one. For example, learning about the illness together, knowing how important it is to take certain medicines, or looking into changes to your lifestyle that can help the illness. This method turns caring for a family member into a learning experience for both the child and the family member.

Bringing everyone together and distributing responsibility:

When kids help with caregiving, building a sense of togetherness and shared duty within the family is very important. This means creating an environment where everyone in the family knows what they can do to help the loved one and gets how much work it takes to deal with the challenges of a chronic sickness.

1. Talks and meetings with family: Hold regular family meetings to discuss how to care for the loved one. Set up a place where kids can talk about their ideas, ask questions, and share what they've seen. This way of working together ensures that everyone is aware of and active in the decisions made, which promotes a sense of shared duty.

2. Setting up a care schedule: Make a care calendar with precise chores and due dates for each family member, including children. This picture shows that caring for someone is an even stronger shared duty. Switch around who is responsible for what so that no one gets too busy and everyone can help with care.

3. Promoting Open Communication: Make it easy for everyone in the family to talk to each other. Kids should feel free to discuss their worries, feelings, and thoughts about caring. Ensure they know you respect their opinions and that what they offer is vital for the family's health.

4. Coming Together to Celebrate Success: Celebrate the successes and goals you and your family have made together. This could be as easy as taking medications as prescribed, starting a new self-care habit, or getting past a specific problem that comes up because of the chronic sickness. Celebrating with your family supports the idea that everyone's work adds up to success.

5. Creating Family traditions: Create family traditions that show unity and shared duty. This could be a family dinner once a week, a set time for sharing stories, or a particular exercise that brings everyone together. These habits make people feel like they belong and support the idea that caring for a loved one is a shared responsibility.

6. Why emotional health is important: When kids are helping with parenting, it's essential to put their mental health first. Some of the feelings kids can have are understanding and compassion, while others may feel sad or frustrated. Their mental growth needs to have a safe place where they can talk about their thoughts and get help.

To sum up, getting kids involved in caring for and supporting a loved one with a long-term illness needs to be done in a way that is thoughtful and proper for their age. Families can make a place where kids can actively contribute to the well-being of a loved one by encouraging a sense of togetherness, shared duty, and open communication. Children learn helpful life skills and kindness, grit, and a deep understanding of how important it is to have family support during hard times.

Chapter 9: How to Answer Questions and Keep People Curious

To build understanding, empathy, and open conversation within the family, it's essential to encourage kids to ask questions about a loved one's long-term sickness. Being patient and honest with them when you answer their questions builds trust and gives you great chances to teach and help them.

Why it's Important to Ask Questions:

Asking kids about a loved one's long-term illness is a great way to help them understand and get rid of any fears or misunderstandings they might have. Kids can learn more, talk about their worries, and be active in the family's journey through dealing with illness when they feel safe enough to say what they're interested in.

1. **"Knowledge gives you power"**: Children learn more about long-term sickness and its effects when encouraged to be curious. When people know more about something, they feel they have more control over it, lowering their worry and giving them a better viewpoint.

2. Putting your worries and feelings into words: Asking questions allows kids to discuss their feelings and concerns. It starts a conversation where they can talk about their feelings, fears, and doubts, which is good for their mental health and gives their family a chance to reassure and help them.

3. Getting people to trust you: Kids and adults can trust each other more when asked questions. When kids know that their questions will be answered honestly and with care, it builds trust and makes them want to keep talking. This trust is essential for making the family relationship open and helpful.

Plans for Dealing with Curiosity

1. Make a safe space: Make sure kids can ask questions without worrying about being judged. Set aside a time for family chats or one-on-one talks so kids can talk about their questions safely.

2. Be patient and listen carefully: When people ask you questions, listen carefully. Let kids say what they're thinking out loud before you answer. This shows that you value their questions, making them more likely to seek answers.

3. Be honest and appropriate for your age: Give real answers that are right for your age. Ensure that information is given clearly and adequately for the child's age and level of growth when you explain things.

4. Draw comparisons and use pictures: Use comparisons or photographs to make complicated medical ideas easier to understand. Children use analogies to connect new words to better understand them to things they already know.

5. Encourage communication that goes both ways: Encourage conversation that goes both ways. Encourage kids to talk about more than just their questions. Let them say what they think and feel. This two-way conversation helps family members understand each other better and strengthens their mental bond.

6. Make people feel normal for being curious: stress that curiosity is a healthy part of learning. It makes it seem normal to ask questions, reinforcing the idea that looking for information is good.

7. Allow them to have a say in decisions: Include kids in decision-making about the proper long-term illness for their age. This not only gives them more power, but it also makes them feel like their opinion is valued in the family.

Sources for materials that are right for kids' ages:

Giving kids age-appropriate materials is essential for helping them understand their loved one's long-term sickness. By using books and other materials made just for different age groups, you can be sure that the information is clear and valuable.

1. **"Why Does Grandma Have a Cane?" by Judy Wong is a book for kids ages 3 to 7:**

Source: "My Family and Me: A Kid's Guide to Living with a Chronic Illness" (Workbook with activities)

2. **For kids between 8 and 12: Book:** "The Sick Bug" by Aimee E. Valle.

Source: "The Kids' Guide to Working Out Conflicts: How to Keep Cool, Stay Safe, and Get Along" written by Miki Bendis and Naomi Drew

Teenagers (13–18 years old): Book: "It's Not the End of the World" by Judy Blume.

Book: "The Chronic Illness Workbook: Strategies and Solutions for Taking Back Your Life" written by Patricia A. Fennell

4. **For families, the book "The Spoon Theory"** by Christine Miserandino is a good resource. It explains

energy control in a way that is easy to understand. The website is KidsHealth (Kids area). Offers health-related articles and films that are good for all ages

In conclusion, A positive and caring way to talk to your family about a loved one's long-term illness is to answer their questions and satisfy their interest. Asking questions, being patient and honest in response, and giving tools that are right for the child's age all help create a supportive family setting where empathy, understanding, and knowledge sharing can grow. Families can deal with the challenges of a chronic illness together by encouraging open conversation. This builds stronger bonds and a solid basis for the whole family's health.

Chapter 10: Making Your Family Strong

Essential Lessons on How to Tell Kids About a Family Member's Long-Term Illness:

Throughout this guide, a few critical lessons have become clear about how best to explain a loved one's long-term illness to children:

1. **Communicating openly and honestly:** It is imperative to communicate openly and honestly. Kids should be encouraged to talk about their feelings, ask questions, and participate actively in conversations about long-term disease. Giving honest and proper explanations for the child's age builds trust and knowledge.

2. **Making information fit different age groups:** Consider the various stages of growth that children are in and tailor your information to them. Simple, concrete answers may help younger kids, while bigger kids can understand more complicated ones. Age-appropriate tasks and tools help kids understand better.

3. **Building Empathy:** Families need to learn to understand each other. Encourage people to see things from different points of view, show empathy, and do things that help people understand each other. Fostering empathy

helps kids understand what their loved ones are going through and makes family bonds stronger.

4. Making a helpful environment: Give kids a safe place to be where they can feel heard, valued, and included. Thank them for what they've done to help with caregiving, include them in decisions when it's acceptable, and enjoy their successes with them. This makes people feel more united and responsible for each other.

5. Dealing with Emotional Problems: Families may face emotional problems that should be recognized and dealt with. Give ideas on how to make a safe space for kids to talk about their feelings and how to have appropriate chats for each age group. Understanding and accepting feelings are important parts of communicating clearly.

Why it's crucial to build resilience as a family:

Getting more substantial as a family is essential for getting through the complex parts of living with a loved one's ongoing sickness. Resilient families have the strength and flexibility to deal with problems, overcome hard times, and grow together. This is why building resilience is so important:

1. Being able to deal with change: Changes are often complex to predict when someone has a chronic illness.

Resilient families can handle these changes by changing their habits and tactics. Being able to change with the times gives people a sense of security.

2. Dealing with doubt: Being resilient helps families deal with the doubt of having a chronic sickness. Families can deal with the unknown, handle stress, and support each other through the ups and downs of the sickness path by learning how to cope.

3. Makes family ties stronger: Being resilient makes family bonds stronger. Taking on problems together builds unity and a sense of mission. Family members can get strength from each other, which helps them see that they are not going through this trip alone.

4. Encourages a Positive attitude: Resilient Families keep a positive attitude by focusing on their strengths and finding answers instead of dwelling on their problems. This positive outlook helps the family work better together, improves mental health, and lessens the effects of things that cause worry.

5. Encourages Open Communication: Resilience helps family members communicate better. Members feel free to share their feelings and ideas, creating a safe space where problems can be discussed and answers can be found together.

Families can get ongoing help and resources:

1. Helpful Groups: Find support groups in your area or online for families with the same kind of long-term illnesses. Sharing your stories with people going through the same things gives you a sense of connection and understanding.

2. Resources for Therapy: You might want to talk to a family therapist or counselor dealing with chronic sickness and family issues. Getting help from a professional can give you valuable ideas and ways to deal with specific problems.

3. Workshops for education: Go to classes or webinars that teach you about things connected to your chronic sickness. These events can give you helpful knowledge, ways to deal with your problems, and chances to meet other families and experts.

4. Services for the community: Look into the community programs and tools to help families with a member with a long-term illness. This could include short-term care, counseling, or training programs to help families.

5. Continued Education: Use reliable sites to learn about long-term sickness. Never stop teaching kids and adults about new treatments, studies, and ways to live healthier lives that can improve their loved one's health.

6. Ways to take care of yourself: Stress how important it is for everyone in the family to take care of themselves. For people who want to be strong enough to help a loved one with a chronic illness, taking care of their own physical and mental health is essential.

7. Websites and discussion boards: Use websites and chat rooms where families can share tools and experiences. Virtually connecting with others gives you a sense of connection and gives you access to a lot of information and help. Families can get through the process of living with a loved one's chronic illness with strength, unity, and a strong spirit by reviewing key lessons, recognizing how important it is to build resilience, and providing ongoing support and resources. Each family member's input, from honest conversation to active involvement, is crucial for strengthening and supporting the family setting.

Conclusion:

We're going on a journey together in this book. The goal of this trip is to help families figure out how to explain a loved one's long-term illness to their children in a way that they can understand. We've looked into the details of communication, mental health, and resilience with care, considering families' unique problems on this road.

The Way Forward:

As this book ends, it's important to remember that the journey doesn't stop here. Having a loved one with a chronic sickness is a long-term process, and each family's road is different. Being committed to communication, understanding, and power over time strengthens it. Families can overcome this with strength and unity if they encourage open communication, offer mental support, and use the tools. Don't forget that you have friends and family. Many families have been through the same things, and their stories, like yours, add to a larger story of strength, love, and resilience. Enjoy the unique trip your family is on, and remember to enjoy the wins and learn from the setbacks. With each step, you build a base of understanding, kindness, and support that will help you get through the complex parts of living with a chronic sickness in a loved one. This eBook should be a help, a friend, and a motivation for your family as they go on their next trip. As you move forward, remember that your strength, love, and dedication will keep you going. Family can overcome, change, and do well together.